UNRAVELING DEMENTIA

A Journey of Understanding and Empowerment

DR KINSLEY BARDE

TABLE OF CONTENTS

UNDERSTANDING DEMENTIA

The neurological disorder known as dementia is a complicated and gradual condition that affects memory, reasoning, behavior, and the capacity to carry out daily tasks. It is typified by a deterioration in cognitive functioning. People may experience difficulties with understanding, communicating, and maintaining their sense of place and time as the illness worsens. Dementia is a syndrome rather than a single disease that results from a number of underlying diseases that harm brain tissue and impair normal brain function. We will delve into the complexities of dementia in this in-depth examination, including its description, kinds, causes, prevalence, and effects on people and society.

Definition of Dementia

Understanding dementia's complex character and identifying the constellation of symptoms that work together to support a diagnosis are essential to defining the illness. Although the most well-known sign of dementia is frequently memory loss, the illness actually includes a wider range of cognitive deficits. Language, judgment, problem-solving, and spatial awareness issues are a few examples of these. Dementia is a progressive condition, meaning that as brain damage mounts, symptoms get worse over time.

The inability of a person to operate independently in daily life due to cognitive deterioration is one of the main diagnostic criteria for dementia. This feature sets dementia apart from typical age-related declines in cognitive function, which can cause moderate forgetfulness but don't seriously hinder daily functioning.

Standardized diagnostic criteria for dementia are provided by the International Classification of Diseases (ICD-10) and the Diagnostic and Statistical Manual of Mental Disorders (DSM-5). These requirements include a substantial impact on social or vocational performance, impairment in at least two cognitive domains, and evidence of cognitive decline from a prior level of functioning.

While the likelihood of having dementia rises with age, it's crucial to remember that dementia is not a normal aspect of aging. Although older folks, especially those over 65, account for the majority of dementia cases, dementia can also strike younger people; this is known as early-onset or young-onset dementia.

Types of Dementia and Their Causes

There are various forms of dementia, each with unique traits, patterns of onset, and underlying causes.

1. Alzheimer's Disease: Accounting for the majority of cases, Alzheimer's disease is the most common type of dementia. The buildup of aberrant protein deposits in the brain, such as tau tangles and beta-amyloid plaques, is what defines it. These proteins cause the gradual deterioration and death of brain cells by interfering with neural communication. Alzheimer's disease usually starts out with little memory loss and works its way up to more severe cognitive deficiencies such trouble speaking, thinking through problems, and staying focused.

2. Vascular Dementia: This is the second most prevalent kind of dementia and is brought on by reduced blood supply to the brain, which is frequently brought on by small artery disease,

strokes, or transient ischemic episodes (TIAs). Depending on the location and extent of the brain injury, vascular dementia can present with a wide range of cognitive symptoms. Difficulties with executive function, attention, and mental speed are typical symptoms. After a stroke, vascular dementia may develop gradually over time or appear unexpectedly.

3. Dementia with Lewy Bodies (DLB): This type of dementia is distinguished by aberrant protein deposits in the brain known as Lewy bodies. Numerous cognitive, motor, and psychiatric disorders are brought on by these deposits, which interfere with normal brain function. Cognitive fluctuations, visual hallucinations, Parkinsonism (abnormal movement), and REM sleep behavior disorder are all possible symptoms of DLB. Diagnosing DLB is difficult since it shares some clinical characteristics with dementia from Parkinson's disease and Alzheimer's disease.

4. Frontotemporal Dementia (FTD): This condition alters behavior, personality, and language by affecting the frontal and temporal lobes of the brain. Early in the course of the disease, FTD frequently manifests as notable behavioral and personality changes, in contrast to Alzheimer's disease, which predominantly impairs memory and other cognitive skills. Primary progressive aphasia (PPA), semantic variant primary progressive aphasia (svPPA), and behavioral variation frontotemporal dementia (bvFTD) are subtypes of frontotemporal dementia (FTD), each with unique clinical characteristics.

5. Additional Causes of Dementia: In addition to the aforementioned ailments or circumstances, traumatic brain damage, Parkinson's disease, Huntington's disease, HIV/AIDS, certain infections, and metabolic abnormalities can also lead to dementia. A traumatic brain injury can result

in chronic traumatic encephalopathy (CTE), a kind of dementia marked by behavioral abnormalities and cognitive impairment. Examples of these injuries include severe concussions and repetitive head traumas. As Parkinson's disease worsens, cognitive function is often impacted in addition to motor symptoms, leading to Parkinson's disease dementia. An genetic neurodegenerative condition called Huntington's disease is marked by gradual irregularities in mobility, cognitive impairment, and psychiatric problems. HIV-associated neurocognitive disorders (HAND), a collection of cognitive abnormalities, can be brought on by HIV/AIDS. Dementia can also result from some infections, such as Wernicke-Korsakoff syndrome and Creutzfeldt-Jakob disease (CJD), and metabolic conditions.

6. Mixed Dementia: The coexistence of many dementia pathologies in the brain is referred to as mixed dementia. People may, for instance, have both vascular pathology and Alzheimer's disease pathology, which would result in a mix of the cognitive symptoms shared by the two diseases. When an older adult has several underlying risk factors, such as diabetes, hypertension, and cardiovascular disease, they are more likely to get mixed dementia.

Comprehending the many forms and origins of dementia is crucial for precise identification, suitable handling, and customized care preparation for those impacted. The distinctive clinical characteristics, course, and treatment concerns of each kind of dementia emphasize the significance of a thorough examination conducted by medical specialists skilled in dementia care. Furthermore, there is hope for better outcomes and a higher quality of life for those who are living with dementia and their family due to continuous research into the underlying causes of dementia and the development of targeted medicines.

Prevalence and Impact

Globally, the incidence of dementia is rising due to an aging population and advances in healthcare that are extending life expectancy. The World Health Organization (WHO) estimates that 50 million people globally have dementia in 2020, and if current trends continue, this figure is expected to nearly quadruple by 2050.

Dementia affects not just the affected individuals but also their families, carers, and society at large. It can be emotionally, physically, and financially taxing to care for someone who has dementia; it also frequently takes a lot of time and money. High levels of stress, despair, and burnout are common among family caregivers, especially as the illness worsens and the caregiving duties are more difficult.

Dementia places a significant financial strain on healthcare systems and society in addition to the emotional and family costs. As the frequency of dementia rises, it will become more expensive to provide care for those who have dementia, including medical attention, long-term care, and support services. The Alzheimer's Association reports that the expense of dementia care worldwide topped $1 trillion USD in 2018 and is expected to increase significantly over the next several decades.

Dementia also has a big impact on healthcare delivery and public health policies. For impacted people and their families to have the best possible outcomes and quality of life, early detection, diagnosis, and management strategies are essential. To address the growing global burden of dementia, research investments are also critical to better understand the underlying causes of dementia, create effective therapies, and investigate prevention strategies.

Dementia is a varied and intricate syndrome that is marked by a gradual deterioration in cognitive abilities. To effectively address the difficulties caused by dementia and improve outcomes for both caregivers and those who are living with the condition, it is imperative to have a thorough understanding of the definition, kinds, causes, prevalence, and effects of dementia. We can work toward a future where dementia is better understood, treated, and eventually prevented via ongoing research, activism, and support.

DEMENTIA'S NEUROBIOLOGY

A complex neurological disease called dementia is characterized by a steady deterioration in cognitive function. Dementia's pathophysiology must be understood in order to improve diagnostic precision, create effective treatments, and understand the neurobiology underlying the disease.

Brain Structure and Function

The brain is a very complex organ made up of billions of neurons connected by synapses to form intricate neural networks that support behavior, emotion, thought, and other vital processes. Multiple pathogenic processes impair the brain's structural and functional integrity in dementia.

The development of aberrant protein aggregates in the brain is a crucial characteristic of many forms of dementia. For instance, beta-amyloid plaques and tau protein tangles, which impede neuronal communication and ultimately cause cell death, build in particular brain regions in Alzheimer's disease. As the condition worsens, these pathological alterations usually start in brain regions like the entorhinal cortex and hippocampal regions that are crucial for memory and cognition before moving to other parts of the brain.

Damage to the blood arteries in the brain that can lead to ischemic lesions, infarcts, and alterations in the white matter is linked to vascular dementia. These vascular anomalies impede the flow of nutrients and oxygen to the brain's tissue, which damages neurons and impairs cognition. The clinical presentation and severity of symptoms associated with vascular dementia are determined by the location and amount of vascular lesions in the brain.

Lewy bodies are aberrant protein deposits that build up in neurons, especially in the cerebral cortex, brainstem, and subcortical areas, in dementia with Lewy bodies (DLB). These Lewy bodies disrupt the signaling of neurotransmitters, including as serotonin, acetylcholine, and dopamine, which results in a variety of DLB-specific cognitive, motor, and mental symptoms.

The brain's frontal and temporal lobes are known to atrophy and degenerate in people with frontotemporal dementia (FTD). Language, behavior regulation, social cognition, and executive function are all influenced by these areas. People with FTD may see changes in their personality, behavior, and language skills as a result of these neural network disruptions.

Pathological Processes

Dementia is caused by a variety of pathogenic mechanisms that combine environmental, cellular, molecular, and hereditary variables. Multiple shared routes have been linked to the neurodegenerative process, however the precise processes differ based on the kind of dementia.

Dementia is primarily caused by neuroinflammation, which is facilitated by activated microglia and astrocytes that emit pro-inflammatory cytokines, chemokines, and reactive oxygen species. Neurodegeneration and inflammation can feed off one other in a feedback loop when chronic inflammation aggravates neuronal damage and speeds up the course of the disease.

In dementia, excitotoxicity—an overabundance of glutamate receptor activation—can result in cell death and brain damage. The principal excitatory neurotransmitter in the brain is glutamate; nevertheless, glutamate signaling dysregulation can lead to neurotoxicity, especially in diseases such as Alzheimer's disease where beta-amyloid buildup impairs calcium homeostasis and synaptic function.

Dementia is also frequently associated with mitochondrial dysfunction, which is typified by reduced oxidative stress, neural susceptibility, and energy generation impairment. Reactive oxygen species produced during regular cellular respiration can cause damage to mitochondria, which are essential for cellular metabolism. A malfunctioning mitochondria exacerbates the neurodegenerative process by causing neuronal dysfunction and death.

A hallmark of many dementias, such as dementia from Parkinson's disease, dementia from Alzheimer's disease, and dementia with Lewy bodies, is abnormal protein aggregation. Beta-amyloid, tau, and alpha-synuclein are examples of misfolded proteins that build up within neurons and impair cellular activity, resulting in synaptic dysfunction, loss of neurons, and cognitive decline. Protease degradation pathways, chaperone proteins, and genetic predisposition are some of the intricate mechanisms that underlie protein misfolding and aggregation.

Diagnostic Instruments and Biomarkers

The diagnosis and treatment of dementia have been completely transformed by developments in neuroimaging and molecular biomarker research, which have made it possible to identify the underlying illness earlier and with more accuracy.

Computed tomography (CT) and magnetic resonance imaging (MRI) are two structural neuroimaging methods that offer comprehensive information about the anatomy of the brain, including atrophy, white matter alterations, and vascular abnormalities. These imaging methods are useful for tracking the course of the disease over time and finding structural abnormalities linked to particular forms of dementia.

Brain activity and metabolism can be seen by functional neuroimaging methods including single-photon emission computed tomography (SPECT) and positron emission tomography (PET). These imaging methods are able to identify dementia-specific alterations in blood flow patterns, neurotransmitter binding, and glucose metabolism. For instance, beta-amyloid plaques in the brain can be seen with amyloid PET imaging, which helps diagnose Alzheimer's disease and guide therapy choices.

Cerebrospinal fluid (CSF) biomarkers measure specific proteins linked to neurodegeneration and inflammation, offering important insights into the underlying pathology of dementia. For instance, elevated levels of tau and phosphorylated tau (p-tau) proteins in the CSF and lower levels of amyloid-beta42 are suggestive of the pathophysiology of Alzheimer's disease. Similarly, dementia with Lewy bodies is linked to higher levels of alpha-synuclein and lower levels of beta-amyloid42 in the CSF.

Blood-based biomarkers are becoming available as non-invasive methods for prognostication and diagnosis of dementia. These biomarkers, which represent underlying disease processes in the brain, include proteins, lipids, metabolites, and genetic markers. Blood-based biomarkers have potential for early dementia detection and monitoring in clinical practice, but they still need to be confirmed and improved.

In summary, intricate interactions between genetic, molecular, cellular, and environmental factors ultimately result in neuronal malfunction and cognitive loss in dementia, which is distinguished by its neurobiology. In order to improve patient outcomes and quality of life, it is imperative to comprehend the underlying pathogenic mechanisms of dementia and create effective treatments, biomarkers, and diagnostic tools. Prolonged investigation into the neurobiology of dementia is promising in terms of finding new targets for treatment and developing precision medicine strategies for this debilitating illness.

CLINICAL MANIFESTATIONS

A complicated syndrome, dementia presents with a range of cognitive, behavioral, and functional abnormalities. Comprehending the clinical presentations of dementia is crucial for precise diagnosis, suitable handling, and customized treatment strategies.

Symptoms of Cognitive Function

One of the main characteristics of dementia is its cognitive symptoms, which are frequently the first and most noticeable indications of the illness. The aforementioned symptoms indicate deficiencies in multiple cognitive domains, such as executive function, language, memory, attention, and visuospatial skills.

One of the most prevalent cognitive signs of dementia, especially Alzheimer's disease, is memory impairment. At least in the early stages of the condition, people may have trouble recalling current events, discussions, or appointments, but their recollections of earlier events may hold up very well. Both short-term and long-term memory are affected, and memory losses usually become more noticeable and widespread as dementia advances.

Dementia frequently causes problems with attention and concentration, which might show up as forgetfulness, distractibility, or trouble focusing during conversations or work. People could find it difficult to keep organized, follow directions, or finish tasks that call for prolonged concentration.

Language impairments can show themselves in a number of ways, such as anomia (difficulty finding words), alexia (slow speech), and aphasia (difficulty understanding spoken or written language). People could struggle to understand long sentences, follow conversations, or express themselves intelligibly.

Problems with higher-order cognitive functions like reasoning, planning, problem-solving, and decision-making are referred to as executive dysfunction. Dementia patients may find it difficult to start and finish work, make wise decisions, or adjust to new circumstances. The ability to function independently and in daily life might be severely hampered by executive dysfunction.

Problems with perception, interpretation, and navigation of the spatial environment are associated with visuospatial deficits. People could struggle to judge distances, identify persons or items they know, or comprehend spatial relationships. Deficits in vision may be a factor in challenges with tasks like operating a vehicle, interpreting maps, or getting dressed on one's own.

It's critical to understand that individual differences in cognitive reserve and brain resilience, as well as the underlying type and stage of the disorder, can all affect the specific cognitive symptoms of dementia.

Behavioral and Psychological Symptoms

Behavioral and psychological symptoms are prevalent indications of dementia that have a substantial effect on the welfare of those who are afflicted and those who are caring for them. Let's examine these symptoms in more detail:

Dementia's behavioral symptoms include a variety of acts and behaviors that might be upsetting, disturbing, or difficult to control. Aggression, restlessness, disinhibition, agitation, and improper social behavior are a few examples of these symptoms. hostility might include verbal or physical hostility directed against others, whereas agitation is characterized by restlessness, pacing, or repetitive movements. When someone with dementia wanders aimlessly and puts oneself in danger, it is called wandering. Disinhibition appears as a loss of impulse control or social inhibitions, which results in actions or remarks that are improper in public.

These behavioral symptoms frequently result from underlying issues like dissatisfaction, perplexity, impaired senses, or unfulfilled desires. Dementia patients may find it difficult to express their demands or may get overwhelmed by their surroundings, which can result in violent outbursts. Unfamiliar surroundings, schedule modifications, or physical discomfort can sometimes cause behavioral problems.

A comprehensive strategy that addresses both the underlying causes and the current behavioral manifestations is necessary to manage the behavioral symptoms of dementia. Behavioral disruptions can be avoided and managed with the use of non-pharmacological therapies such routine routines, environmental changes, and behavioral therapy approaches. Pharmacological therapies might be taken into consideration in some circumstances, but they should only be used sparingly and under the supervision of medical professionals due to their potential negative effects and limited effectiveness.

Dementia-related psychological symptoms include dysregulation of mood, affect, and emotions. Apathy, impatience, anxiety, and depression are typical psychological symptoms. Dementia patients may exhibit a range of emotional expressions, from agitation and restlessness to grief and despair. Apathy, which is defined as a lack of interest or drive, is very prevalent among dementia patients and has a substantial negative influence on their participation in day-to-day activities.

Psychological symptoms can worsen functional decline and cognitive impairments, significantly impairing an individual's independence and quality of life. A comprehensive strategy that takes into account the interactions between biological, psychological, and social components is necessary to address psychological symptoms. Supportive counseling, cognitive-behavioral therapy, and mindfulness-based interventions are a few examples of psychosocial interventions that can help people manage their emotional discomfort and enhance their general well-being.

Delusions and hallucinations are examples of psychotic symptoms that are rather common in some dementia types, such as dementia with Lewy bodies and dementia from Parkinson's disease. Perceiving non-realistic sensory experiences, such as seeing or hearing things that aren't there, is known as hallucinations. Fixed incorrect beliefs that are unaffected by logic or evidence are called delusions. For those suffering from dementia, these psychotic symptoms can be upsetting and may even be a factor in behavioral issues and caregiver stress.

A person's mood, general well-being, and ability to think clearly can all be significantly impacted by sleep difficulties, which are also common in dementia patients. Sundowning, or heightened disorientation and agitation in the late afternoon or evening, excessive daytime sleepiness, insomnia (difficulty falling or staying asleep), and restless legs syndrome are examples of sleep disruptions. A multidisciplinary strategy is necessary to address sleep disruptions in dementia patients and their caregivers. This approach should address underlying medical disorders, environmental variables, and behavioral interventions to encourage good sleep patterns and improve the quality of sleep.

To sum up, behavioral and psychological symptoms are prevalent indications of dementia that have a substantial influence on the well-being of both the afflicted person and their carers. In order to effectively address these symptoms, a complete strategy that takes into account the underlying reasons, unique needs, and preferences of each person with dementia must be implemented. Caregivers must also be given the support and tools they need to successfully navigate these difficulties. Individuals suffering from dementia can enhance their quality of life and preserve their dignity and autonomy while managing the intricacies of the illness by attending to their behavioral and psychological symptoms.

Functional Decline and Impairment

As dementia advances, major obstacles for those affected include functional decline and limitations. Let's look more closely at this subject:

People with dementia frequently see a decline in their ability to do instrumental activities of daily living (IADLs) and activities of daily living (ADLs) as their dementia progresses. ADLs include basic self-care activities including clothing, bathing, using the restroom, grooming, and feeding that are necessary for maintaining physical and personal hygiene. IADLs, on the other hand, include more intricate tasks like handling money, cooking, shopping, and using transit that are required for independent living in the community.

Cognitive, physical, sensory, and behavioral deficits all contribute to the progressive functional deterioration seen in dementia. Individuals with cognitive abnormalities, including executive dysfunction, memory loss, and visuospatial impairments, may find it more difficult to plan, organize, and complete daily chores. For instance, a person suffering from dementia can become confused when attempting to traverse their home or forget how to brush their teeth.

Movement and coordination issues are a result of physical limitations such as balance issues, gait abnormalities, and motor deficits. Dementia increases the risk of falls and accidents in those who struggle to move, transition from one surface to another, or maintain balance. Their independence and functional abilities are further compromised by these physical constraints.

Sensory impairments that worsen functional impairments and safety issues include deficiencies in vision or hearing. Uncertainty about depth perception or trouble identifying things due to visual agnosia are examples of visual disturbances that might impair one's ability to appropriately perceive their surroundings. Similar to how hearing loss can make it harder for a person to comprehend spoken instructions or communicate socially, hearing loss can further isolate a person and make it more difficult for them to go about their everyday lives.

Individuals with dementia become more dependent on caregivers for basic needs and safety monitoring as their functional decline advances. Along with helping with meal preparation, medicine administration, and transportation, caregivers may need to offer direct support with activities like dressing, bathing, and using the restroom. Being a caregiver may be physically and mentally taxing, especially if the severity of care needs to rise as a disease progresses.

One of the main objectives of care for people with dementia is to preserve their independence and quality of life. A variety of interventions can assist in promoting functional capacities and autonomy. The goal of occupational therapy is to increase a person's capacity to carry out ADLs and IADLs by using strategies such task simplification, adaptive equipment, and environment adjustments. Enhancing mobility, strength, and balance is the goal of physical therapy in order to lower the risk of falls and preserve functional independence. Installing grab bars, handrails, and non-slip flooring, for example, can make a home safer for those who are living with dementia.

Dementia patients' everyday lives are profoundly impacted by functional decline and impairments, which hinder their capacity to carry out necessary duties and preserve their independence. A comprehensive strategy that takes into account the complex nature of dementia and includes therapies to promote cognitive, physical, sensory, and behavioral function is needed to address these issues. Individuals with dementia can maximize their functional abilities and quality of life with customized care and support, and caregivers can get the help and resources they require to successfully manage the caring journey.

In conclusion, a wide range of cognitive, behavioral, and functional abnormalities that affect a person's capacity to think, act, and do daily tasks are included in the clinical manifestations of dementia. In order to provide comprehensive care, maximize quality of life, and promote the wellbeing of people with dementia and their families, it is imperative to comprehend and manage these manifestations. Individuals suffering from dementia can receive the individualized treatment and assistance they require to manage the difficulties of this complicated condition by means of a multidisciplinary strategy that incorporates medical, psychological, and supporting therapies.

IDENTIFICATION AND EVALUATION OF DEMENTIA

Dementia diagnosis entails a thorough assessment of behavioral, cognitive, and functional symptoms in addition to taking into account the patient's medical history, physical examination results, and results of diagnostic testing. For proper management, treatment planning, and support for dementia patients and their carers, an accurate diagnosis is crucial.

Diagnostic Criteria

Standardized criteria developed by medical organizations, such as the International Classification of Diseases (ICD-10) and the Diagnostic and Statistical Manual of Mental Disorders (DSM-5) guide the diagnosis of dementia. The following criteria list the essential characteristics and diagnostic standards for dementia:

- Historical, clinical, and/or neuropsychological testing evidence of cognitive deterioration from a prior level of functioning.
- Deficit in a minimum of two cognitive areas, including language, attention, executive function, memory, and visuospatial skills.
- A notable functional deterioration brought on by cognitive impairment in ADLs and/or IADLs, or instrumental activities of daily living.
- Symptoms that cannot be attributed to substance abuse, mental illnesses, or other medical ailments.

Based on particular clinical characteristics and diagnostic indicators, the DSM-5 also outlines criteria for several subtypes of dementia, including Lewy body dementia, Alzheimer's disease, vascular dementia, and frontotemporal dementia.

A comprehensive clinical history that covers the beginning and course of symptoms, co-occurring conditions, medication usage, family history, and functional status is usually part of the diagnostic evaluation process. To check for indications of neurological, vascular, or other systemic disorders that could exacerbate cognitive impairment, a physical examination may also be performed.

To systematically evaluate cognitive function and identify minor deficits in language, attention, memory, visuospatial ability, and executive function, neuropsychological testing is frequently used. Neuropsychological assessments can offer significant insights into the nature and extent of cognitive impairments, supporting both differential diagnosis and therapy strategizing.

Diagnostic imaging tests, including computed tomography (CT) and magnetic resonance imaging (MRI), can be used to check for structural abnormalities in the brain, such as lesions, atrophy, infarcts, and changes in the white matter. Neuroimaging can be used to rule out other explanations for cognitive decline and can offer proof in favor of certain dementias, such Alzheimer's or vascular dementia.

Tests for biomarkers, such as the analysis of cerebrospinal fluid (CSF) and molecular imaging (PET, for example), can be used to look for pathological processes that may be underlying dementia, such as tau protein abnormalities, neuroinflammation, and beta-amyloid deposition. The differentiation of dementia subgroups and the prediction of disease progression are two areas in which biomarker testing is especially helpful.

Distinctive Diagnosis

In order to differentiate dementia from other medical problems, psychiatric disorders, and reversible causes of cognitive impairment, differential diagnosis is crucial. The following common conditions can mimic dementia:

- Delirium: Acute confusional state with a fast onset, erratic course, trouble paying attention, and altered consciousness. Delirium is treatable with the right care and can be brought on by a number of illnesses, drugs, or environmental triggers.

- Mild cognitive impairment (MCI): An intermediate stage between dementia and normal aging, marked by objective cognitive impairment on neuropsychological tests and subjective cognitive complaints; however, functional independence is maintained, and there is no discernible impairment in daily living activities.

- Depression: A mood condition marked by enduring melancholy, hopelessness, and loss of interest in or enjoyment from activities; it is frequently accompanied by cognitive symptoms such memory problems, reduced attention, and indecision. In the differential diagnosis of dementia, depression should be taken into account as it might resemble cognitive impairment in older persons.

- Normal age-related cognitive changes: Memory loss, processing speed reductions, and cognitive elasticity are all prevalent as people age and may not always signify dementia. Nonetheless, behavioral abnormalities, functional deterioration, or notable impairment across several cognitive domains should raise the possibility of underlying dementia.

- Neurological disorders: Cognitive impairment, movement symptoms, or other neurological aspects that may overlap with dementia can be present in conditions including Parkinson's disease, Huntington's disease, multiple sclerosis, and normal pressure hydrocephalus. A comprehensive neurological assessment that looks at motor function, reflexes, and gait can help distinguish these disorders from dementia.

- Metabolic and endocrine disorders: In the differential diagnosis of dementia, hypothyroidism, vitamin B12 insufficiency, hypercalcemia, and metabolic disturbances should all be taken into account as potential causes of cognitive impairment. Cognitive symptoms may be caused by underlying metabolic or endocrine disorders, which can be found and treated with the aid of laboratory tests.

- Substance-related disorders: Cognitive function can be impaired and dementia mimicked by long-term alcoholism, substance misuse, and prescription side effects. Assessing cognitive symptoms and choosing the best course of action requires a thorough history of substance use, including the use of alcohol and prescription medications.

A comprehensive clinical assessment that includes a patient's medical history, physical examination, cognitive testing, laboratory tests, and diagnostic imaging scans is necessary to distinguish dementia from its imitators. To obtain an accurate diagnosis and create a thorough treatment plan, healthcare specialists from a variety of disciplines—including neurologists, psychiatrists, geriatricians, and neuropsychologists—often collaborate multidisciplinaryly.

Comprehensive Evaluation Methods

In order to evaluate the cognitive, functional, and psychosocial needs of people with dementia and customize therapies to meet those needs, comprehensive assessment procedures are crucial. These methods generally entail a multidisciplinary assessment conducted by a group of medical specialists, such as doctors, nurses, social workers, occupational therapists, and neuropsychologists, who have experience with dementia care.

A complete clinical history that covers the origin and course of cognitive symptoms, medical comorbidities, medication usage, and psychosocial factors is usually the first step in a full examination. Insights regarding behavioral, emotional, and functional changes as well as the person's social support system and care requirements can be obtained from family members and caregivers.

To look for indications of neurological, vascular, or other systemic disorders that could lead to cognitive impairment, a physical examination is conducted. To identify potential areas of concern and direct additional assessment and management, vital signs, neurological status, sensory function, gait and balance, and overall functional status are assessed.

A key component of a thorough evaluation for dementia is neuropsychological testing, which offers objective measurements of cognitive function in a variety of areas, such as language, memory, attention, and visuospatial ability, as well as executive function. Neuropsychological assessments evaluate cognitive abilities and limitations, spot impairment patterns, and direct the development and tracking of treatment plans.

An individual's capacity to carry out instrumental activities of daily living (IADLs) and activities of daily living (ADLs) on their own is assessed through a functional assessment. Basic self-care activities like washing, dressing, using the restroom, grooming, and feeding fall under the category of ADLs, but more complicated duties like handling money, cooking, grocery shopping, and traveling are included in IADLs. In order to maximize independence and quality of life, therapies that target areas of functional decline are informed by the results of functional assessments.

An individual's social support system, caregiver load, and psychological requirements are assessed through psychosocial assessment. When evaluating the individual's psychosocial environment and creating a thorough care plan, factors such as family dynamics, caregiver stress, financial resources, stable housing, and accessibility to community support services are taken into account. An essential part of dementia care is psychosocial interventions, which should be customized to the requirements of the patient and caregiver. These interventions include caregiver education, support groups, respite care, and community services.

In summary, a complete strategy integrating clinical examination, cognitive testing, functional assessment, and psychosocial evaluation is necessary for the diagnosis and assessment of dementia. Eliminating other possible reasons of cognitive impairment, such as delirium, depression, mild cognitive impairment, and neurological or metabolic problems, is necessary for an accurate diagnosis. For the purpose of directing treatment decisions, creating individualized care plans, and maximizing outcomes for dementia patients and their carers, differential diagnosis and thorough assessment are crucial. Throughout the course of the disease, thorough, holistic care must be provided to individuals with dementia, which requires multidisciplinary teamwork among healthcare specialists to fulfill their unique demands.

TREATMENT MODALITIES

Cognitive decline and functional disability are hallmarks of dementia, an advancing and incurable disorder. Although there isn't a cure for dementia at this time, there are a number of treatment options that can help patients and their carers manage symptoms, maximize functional abilities, and improve quality of life. Treatment modalities that are customized to each patient's needs and preferences usually include non-pharmacological therapies, pharmaceutical interventions, and multimodal methods.

Drug-Related Interventions

The main goals of pharmacological therapies for dementia are to treat the underlying pathological processes linked to particular forms of dementia, manage behavioral issues, and lessen cognitive symptoms. The following drugs are frequently prescribed to treat dementia:

- Cholinesterase Inhibitors: Galantamine, rivastigmine, and donepezil are examples of cholinesterase inhibitors that are authorized for the treatment of mild to moderate Alzheimer's disease. Acetylcholine is a neurotransmitter that is involved in memory and cognitive function; these drugs act by boosting its availability in the brain. In patients with Alzheimer's disease, cholinesterase inhibitors may help reduce cognitive symptoms, slow the illness's progression, and improve general functioning.

The N-methyl-D-aspartate (NMDA) receptor antagonist memantine is authorized for the management of mild to severe Alzheimer's disease. Memantine reduces excitotoxicity and neuronal damage linked to dementia by modulating glutamate neurotransmission. When combined with cholinesterase inhibitors, memantine may help people with moderate to severe Alzheimer's disease reduce behavioral abnormalities, stabilize functional abilities, and improve cognitive symptoms.

- Antipsychotic Drugs: People with dementia who exhibit behavioral abnormalities such as agitation, hostility, and psychosis may be prescribed antipsychotic drugs such risperidone, olanzapine, and quetiapine. Antipsychotic drugs should, however, be used with caution due to their potential for side effects, which include drowsiness, extrapyramidal symptoms, metabolic disruptions, and an increased risk of death, especially in older people with psychosis connected to dementia.

- Antidepressant Drugs: People with dementia may be administered antidepressant drugs, such as serotonin-norepinephrine reuptake inhibitors (SNRIs) and selective serotonin reuptake inhibitors (SSRIs), to treat their symptoms of anxiety and depression. Antidepressants can help elevate mood, lessen agitation, and increase general wellbeing; nevertheless, they should be used with caution and side effects closely watched, especially in older persons with dementia and co-occurring medical disorders.

- Symptomatic medications: To address particular behavioral problems in dementia patients, case-by-case consideration may be given to symptomatic medications such as anticonvulsants for agitation, stimulants for apathy, and benzodiazepines for anxiety. However, especially in older patients with dementia and many comorbidities, these drugs should be administered carefully and thoroughly monitored for potential dangers, drug interactions, and bad effects.

Under the supervision of medical specialists skilled in dementia care, pharmacological therapies ought to be started, followed up on, and modified while considering the needs, preferences, and risk factors of each patient. For people with dementia, regular medication reviews, dose modifications, and side effect monitoring are crucial to maximizing treatment results and reducing any possible dangers related to pharmacotherapy.

Non-Pharmacological Interventions

Non-pharmacological interventions are essential to the management of dementia and are advised as initial treatments for behavioral, cognitive, and functional symptoms. They also help to enhance the quality of life for both the carer and the person suffering from dementia. Non-pharmacological therapies comprise a broad spectrum of techniques, such as:

- Cognitive Stimulation: Activities that aim to engage people with dementia in meaningful and stimulating activities to enhance cognitive function, promote social interaction, and maintain cognitive reserve include reminiscence therapy, reality orientation, memory training, and cognitive games. Cognitive stimulation programs can be customized to each person's interests and skills and given either individually or in a group setting.

- Physical Activity: Research has demonstrated that physical activity therapies, such as aerobic exercise, strength training, balancing exercises, and flexibility exercises, enhance cognitive function, mood, and general physical health in dementia patients. Frequent exercise can improve neuroplasticity, cardiovascular fitness, and lower the incidence of falls and functional deterioration in dementia patients.

- Occupational Therapy: The goal of occupational therapy interventions is to maximize a person's capacity to carry out instrumental activities of daily living (IADLs) and activities of daily living (ADLs) on their own. In order to address deficiencies in motor skills, executive function, and environmental adaption, occupational therapists evaluate their patients' functional capacities, pinpoint obstacles to independence, and create individualized interventions.

- Speech and Language Therapy: Interventions in speech and language therapy are intended to treat communication problems in dementia patients, such as dysarthria, aphasia, and pragmatic language deficits. Speech therapists evaluate people's communication skills, offer verbal and nonverbal communication improvement techniques, and assist carers in fostering productive conversations with those who have dementia.

- Music Therapy: To improve mood, lessen agitation, and increase social engagement in dementia patients, music therapy therapies employ music-based activities such singing, playing instruments, listening to music, and engaging in rhythmic movement. Even in the most advanced stages of the disease, music therapy can elicit emotional reactions, stimulate cognitive performance, and foster relaxation and overall well-being in dementia patients.

- Sensory Stimulation: To engage people with dementia and encourage relaxation, memories, and emotional regulation, sensory stimulation interventions make use of sensory-rich surroundings, multisensory stimuli, and sensory-based activities. Depending on the preferences and sensory requirements of the individual, sensory stimulation activities can include things like aromatherapy, tactile stimulation, multisensory rooms, and therapeutic gardens.

Individualized, person-centered, and culturally sensitive non-pharmacological therapies that include each person's preferences, talents, and specific requirements are necessary. To identify suitable non-pharmacological interventions, set realistic goals, and track progress over time, collaborative care planning involving individuals with dementia, caregivers, and healthcare professionals is necessary.

Multimodal Methods

Pharmacological and non-pharmacological interventions are integrated in multimodal methods to dementia management in order to address cognitive, functional, and behavioral symptoms holistically and maximize treatment outcomes for both dementia patients and their carers. Multimodal treatments strive to improve overall quality of life by addressing various domains of functioning at once, acknowledging the complex and diverse character of dementia.

Pharmacotherapy side effects can be minimized, dependence on medicine can be decreased, and treatment efficacy can be increased by combining pharmaceutical and non-pharmacological therapies. For instance, cholinesterase inhibitors or memantine combined with physical activity, cognitive stimulation, and occupational therapy may have synergistic benefits that improve the general well-being, cognitive performance, and functional independence of people with dementia.

To address the psychosocial needs of people with dementia and their caregivers, multimodal approaches may also include psychosocial therapies, caregiver support, and community services. Better outcomes for people with dementia and their families can be achieved by providing education, counseling, and support groups for caregivers. These interventions can also help reduce caregiver burden, strengthen coping mechanisms, and increase caregiver resilience.

The degree of the disease, the kind of dementia, comorbidities, and personal preferences are among the individual aspects that determine how effective multimodal methods to dementia management are. Essential elements of multimodal dementia care include individualized treatment regimens, ongoing treatment response monitoring, and necessary intervention adjustments.

There are several ways to treat dementia, including non-pharmacological, multimodal, and pharmaceutical techniques that are customized to each patient's needs and preferences. Non-pharmacological interventions are essential for boosting cognitive function, encouraging functional independence, and enhancing quality of life for people with dementia and their carers. While pharmaceutical interventions may help manage behavioral disturbances and reduce cognitive symptoms, non-pharmacological interventions are critical for improving cognitive symptoms. A comprehensive and all-encompassing approach to managing dementia is provided by multimodal approaches that combine pharmaceutical and non-pharmacological interventions. This approach addresses the complex and multifaceted nature of dementia and maximizes treatment outcomes for affected individuals and their families.

CAREGIVING STRATEGIES

Providing dementia care for a loved one may be gratifying as well as difficult. Caregivers may have a wide range of practical, psychological, and physical difficulties as the illness worsens, which may have an adverse influence on their health and capacity to deliver quality care. Effective caregiving for people with dementia requires an understanding of the obstacles faced by the caregiver, the development of coping skills, and the use of support networks.

Understanding Caregiver Challenges

Providing care for an individual suffering from dementia poses distinct obstacles that change as the illness progresses. Among the major difficulties caregivers encounter are:

- Cognitive and Behavioral Symptoms: People suffering from dementia may display confusion, agitation, anger, wandering, memory loss, and hallucinations, among other cognitive and behavioral symptoms. It can be difficult to manage these symptoms, and caregivers may need to exercise patience, ingenuity, and flexibility.

- Communication Difficulties: Language difficulties, comprehension deficiencies, and trouble expressing thoughts and feelings are all major causes of communication breakdowns in dementia. In order to promote productive engagement, caregivers may need to modify their communication style in light of the challenges they may face in comprehending the needs and preferences of persons suffering from dementia.

- Functional Decline: People with dementia endure a progressive loss of functioning as well as impairments in their ability to do instrumental activities of daily living (IADLs) and activities of daily living (ADLs). When it comes to activities like dressing, bathing, using the restroom, grooming, preparing meals, managing medications, and traveling, caregivers may need to offer more support and monitoring.

- Caregiver Stress and Burnout: Providing physical, emotional, and financial support to a person suffering from dementia can be taxing on the caregiver, resulting in stress, burnout, and caregiver burden. While navigating the difficulties of caregiving and witnessing the decline of their loved one, caregivers may feel guilty, angry, frustrated, and grieved.

- Social Isolation: Taking on caregiving tasks might interfere with a caregiver's leisure and social life, which can cause them to withdraw from their friends, family, and community. Stress and feelings of isolation may be exacerbated for caregivers if they experience loneliness, lack of support, and social disconnection.

- Financial Strain: Providing care for an individual with dementia can place a heavy financial load on carers, since they may have to pay for medical treatment, prescription drugs, home adaptations, assistive technology, and caregiving services themselves. Complex financial and legal matters, such as guardianship, Medicaid eligibility, long-term care insurance, and estate planning, may need to be negotiated by caregivers.

To effectively address caregivers' needs and promote their well-being throughout the caregiving journey, it is imperative to recognize and comprehend these caregiver obstacles.

Support Networks and Coping Strategies

Support networks and coping strategies are essential for assisting caregivers in managing the difficulties of providing care for a person with dementia while also preserving their own mental and physical health. Among the coping strategies and networks of support available to caregivers are:

- Self-Care: In order to properly care for their loved ones who have dementia, caregivers must put their own health and well-being first. Caregivers can reduce stress and enhance general well-being by exercising regularly, eating healthily, getting adequate sleep, and using stress-reduction strategies including deep breathing exercises, mindfulness meditation, and relaxation techniques.

- Seeking Social Support: Professional organizations that specialize in dementia care, friends, family, and support groups are all excellent places for caregivers to look for social support. Making connections with other caregivers who are aware of their struggles and experiences can offer support, understanding, and useful tips for managing the stress of caregiving.

- Setting Realistic Expectations: Caregivers should be aware of the limitations of their role as caregivers and seek assistance when necessary in order to create realistic expectations for both themselves and their loved ones who are suffering from dementia. By accepting assistance from friends, family, and local resources, caregivers can lessen their workload and avoid burnout.

- Respite Care: By providing expert assistance and supervision for individuals with dementia, respite care services offer temporary relief for caregivers, enabling them to take breaks, tend to their own needs, and rejuvenate. Numerous options exist for providing respite care, such as adult day programs, in-home respite, overnight respite stays, and residential respite facilities.

- Professional Counseling: Therapists and counselors with a background in counseling can offer caregivers coping mechanisms, emotional support, and techniques for handling stress, bereavement, and caregiver load. Caregivers might benefit from individual therapy, support groups, and caregiver education programs to learn appropriate coping strategies and manage the range of emotions that come with providing care.

- Caregiver Education and Training: Programs for caregivers equip them with the information, tools, and practical skills they need to handle the day-to-day difficulties of providing care for a person suffering from dementia. Communication methods, behavior control plans, safety measures, and self-care routines are a few possible topics.

Long-Term Planning and Respite Care

Effective caregiving for people with dementia requires both long-term planning and respite care, which support carers in managing their obligations and making future plans. Caretakers who receive respite care can take short breaks, tend to their personal needs, and avoid burnout. Making decisions on care alternatives, finances, legal matters, and end-of-life desires is all part of long-term planning. Important factors for long-term planning and respite care include:

- Determining Respite Care Options: Caregivers should investigate the many forms of respite care offered in their neighborhood, such as adult day programs, in-home services, overnight respite stays, and residential respite facilities. When choosing respite care providers, caregivers ought to take their loved one's requirements, preferences, and safety into account.

- Emergency Situation Planning: In the event of an illness, hospital stay, or caregiver disability, caregivers should create backup plans. Caregivers can have peace of mind and continuity of care by having a backup plan in place and communicating critical information to friends, family, and healthcare providers.

- Talking About Long-Term Care Preferences: Caregivers should be upfront and honest with their loved ones about their preferences for home care, assisted living, memory care, and nursing home care, among other forms of long-term care. Dementia patients can express their values and intentions for medical care, end-of-life care, and surrogate decision-making through advance care planning.

- Legal and Financial Planning: When it comes to significant legal and financial issues, such as Medicaid planning, long-term care insurance, advance directives, guardianship, estate planning, power of attorney, and asset protection techniques, caregivers should speak with legal and financial experts. Caretakers who plan ahead can guarantee that their loved ones' future demands are satisfied and successfully handle challenging legal and financial situations.

- Using Community Resources: Caregivers should make use of the community resources and support services that are offered to people with dementia and their carers. These services and resources include adult day centers, caregiver education workshops, adult support groups, and helplines. Making connections with neighborhood organizations, nonprofits, and advocacy groups that focus on dementia care can give caregivers access to helpful resources, support, and recommendations.

In conclusion, caring for a person who has dementia has special obstacles that necessitate the development of useful coping strategies and the utilization of support networks in order to preserve the caregiver's personal wellbeing and deliver high-quality care for their loved ones. Effective caregiving for people with dementia and their carers requires grasping the difficulties faced by caregivers, reaching out for social support, putting self-care first, obtaining respite care, and making long-term plans. Throughout the caring journey, caregivers may improve the quality of life for themselves and their loved ones with dementia by attending to their needs and building their resilience.

ETHICAL AND LEGAL CONSIDERATION

Providing care for people suffering from dementia has distinct moral and legal obstacles with decision-making, self-governance, agreement, and terminal illness management. While legal frameworks create rights, safeguards, and processes for both those with dementia and their caregivers, dementia care is provided in accordance with ethical values such as respect for autonomy, beneficence, non-maleficence, and justice.

Making Informed Decisions and Consent

Fundamental ethical concepts in dementia care include informed consent and decision-making ability, which guarantee that people with dementia are as much as possible involved in decisions about their care and treatment. But as dementia progresses, it can become more difficult to make decisions, which makes substitute decision-making and informed consent difficult. When deciding what to do and giving informed consent to someone who has dementia, important moral and legal factors to take into account are:

Evaluating Decision-Making Capacity: It is the duty of healthcare practitioners to evaluate a person's capacity for making decisions, which includes their comprehension of pertinent information, awareness of the implications of their choices, and ability to express their preferences. Given the erratic character of cognitive function in dementia, capacity evaluations must to be carried out in a courteous and supportive manner.

- Shared Decision Making: In order to investigate treatment alternatives, weigh advantages and risks, and come to an agreement on care objectives and preferences, healthcare professionals, people with dementia, and their caregivers collaborate in shared decision making talks. Informed choices and patient-centered care are promoted through shared decision making, which also respects people's autonomy and values.

- Advance Care Planning: Through advance care planning, people suffering from dementia can communicate their desires and wishes for future medical care, end-of-life care, and surrogate decision-making. Advance directives serve as legal records of people's preferences and serve as a guide for healthcare decision-making in the event that people are unable to make decisions for themselves. Examples of advance directives include living wills, healthcare proxies, and do-not-resuscitate orders.

- Surrogate Decision Making: In situations where people suffering from dementia are unable to make decisions for themselves, family members, guardians, or healthcare proxies may act as surrogate decision makers and make decisions on their behalf in accordance with their known preferences, values, and best interests. It is the fiduciary duty of surrogate decision makers to act in the person's best interests and honor their previously communicated desires.

- Ethical Dilemmas: When a person's preferences, values, and best interests collide with the law, medical advice, or family dynamics, an ethical challenge in dementia care may occur. In order to reach morally sound decisions, ethical decision makers must carefully weigh the conflicting interests and values at issue while striking a balance between the principles of autonomy, beneficence, non-maleficence, and justice.

End-of-life Care and Advanced Directives

It is important to carefully examine the desires, values, and quality of life preferences of individuals with dementia, as well as the ethical and legal guidelines pertaining to autonomy, dignity, and comfort, when providing end-of-life care. Living wills and healthcare proxies are examples of advanced directives that are essential for directing end-of-life decision making and guaranteeing that people's wishes are honored. Important factors to take into account when providing advanced directives and end-of-life care for dementia patients are:

- Palliative Care: This type of care aims to improve the quality of life for patients with advanced dementia and their families by addressing pain, symptom relief, and other related issues. Palliative care emphasizes comfort, dignity, and comprehensive support throughout the course of the disease. It attends to the physical, emotional, and spiritual needs of the patient.

- Hospice Care: Those with advanced dementia who have a finite amount of time left to live—typically six months or less—can get specialized end-of-life care through hospice care. Hospice services can be provided in-home or in a hospice center, and they include pain management, symptom control, emotional support, and spiritual care.

- Withholding and Withdrawing Treatment: When providing end-of-life care for dementia patients, ethical and legal issues pertaining to the withholding and withdrawal of life-sustaining treatments, such as artificial nutrition and hydration, mechanical ventilation, and cardiopulmonary resuscitation, may come up. It is imperative for healthcare practitioners and surrogate decision makers to weigh the advantages and disadvantages of medical measures while honoring patients' desires for their final hours of life.

- Family Dynamics and Conflict Resolution: When making end-of-life decisions for a person with dementia, family dynamics and conflicts might come up, especially if there are disagreements among family members about treatment options, care objectives, and advance directives. The use of ethical consultations, family meetings, and mediation can help to settle disagreements, improve communication, and come to a decision about care that respects the person's preferences and best interests.

- Bereavement Support: After a loved one with dementia passes away, caregivers and family members need to get bereavement support programs. Individuals can express their emotions, share their experiences, and receive support from others who have suffered similar losses through grief counseling, support groups, and memorial services.

Legal Rights and Protection for People Experiencing Dementia

Enshrined in national and international laws, rules, and recommendations that strive to protect the autonomy, dignity, and well-being of people with dementia are legal rights and protections. Procedures for guardianship, advance care planning, surrogate decision-making, and abuse and exploitation prevention are outlined in legal frameworks. Important legal rights and safeguards for those suffering from dementia include:

- Right to Informed Consent: People who have dementia have the right to understandable information regarding their diagnosis, prognosis, available treatments, dangers, and benefits. When it is feasible, healthcare providers have a moral and legal duty to seek informed permission from dementia patients, respecting their autonomy and ability for decision-making.

- Right to Dignity and Respect: Regardless of their functional limits or cognitive ability, people with dementia have the right to be treated with dignity, respect, and compassion. Healthcare professionals should support people's well-being and quality of life throughout the course of a condition while respecting their right to privacy, autonomy, and sense of self.

- Right to Self-Determination: To the degree that they are capable, people with dementia have the right to make decisions regarding their own lives, including those regarding their care, housing, and end-of-life care. Planning for advance care enables people to fulfill their right to self-determination by stating their preferences and wants before they become incapacitated.

- Legal Protections from Abuse and Exploitation: Because of their cognitive deficits and reliance on others for care, people with dementia are susceptible to abuse, neglect, and exploitation. Legal safeguards such as guardianship laws, adult protective services, and reporting requirements for elder abuse are designed to protect people with dementia from harm and to guarantee their safety and well-being.

- Right to Legal Representation: To safeguard their rights, speak out for their interests, and make sure that their desires and wishes are honored, people with dementia have the right to legal representation. For those who lack the capacity to make decisions for themselves and need surrogate decision makers to act on their behalf in financial and legal affairs, legal guardianship may be required.

In summary, informed consent, decision-making ability, end-of-life care, advanced directives, and legal rights and protections for dementia patients are all ethical and legal factors to be taken into account when providing care for those with the disease. It is the joint duty of healthcare providers, caregivers, and family members to follow moral standards, honor people's autonomy and dignity, and make sure their rights are upheld all the way through a disease's course. It is possible for stakeholders to advance person-centered care, improve quality of life, and protect the rights and dignity of individuals with dementia by incorporating ethical and legal frameworks into dementia care practices.

RESEARCH DEVELOPMENTS AND UPCOMING PATHS

Recent years have seen a tremendous advancement in the study of dementia thanks to developments in neuroscience, genetics, technology, and interdisciplinary cooperation. This advancement has resulted in a better comprehension of the fundamental causes of dementia, the discovery of new therapeutic targets, and the creation of creative treatments meant to stop, postpone, or treat the illness. This section will examine the state of dementia research at the moment, possible treatment targets, and new developments in dementia research.

Present-day Research Environment

A wide range of studies examining several facets of dementia, such as its origin, pathophysiology, risk factors, diagnosis, treatment, and prevention, characterize the state of dementia research today. Important study areas include of:

- Genetics and Genomics: Research in these fields has revealed a wide range of genetic susceptibility genes and risk factors linked to dementia, including frontotemporal dementia, Alzheimer's disease, and other neurodegenerative illnesses. Common and uncommon genetic variations raising the risk of dementia have been found using genome-wide association studies (GWAS), whole-exome sequencing, and genome-wide linkage analyses. These findings offer new perspectives on the mechanisms underlying the disease and suggest possible targets for treatment.

- Diagnostic Tools and Biomarkers: Biomarkers are essential for the early identification, diagnosis, and surveillance of dementia. They enable the more precise identification of individuals who are at risk and the tracking of the disease's progression over time. A few examples of biomarkers are blood-based indicators (like plasma amyloid and neurofilament light), genetic markers (like the APOE genotype), cerebrospinal fluid (CSF) proteins (like amyloid-beta, tau, and neurofilament light), and neuroimaging measurements (like amyloid PET, tau PET, and MRI). Promising developments in biomarker research could help with early intervention, tracking treatment response, and more for dementia patients.

The intricate mechanisms driving neuronal malfunction, synapse loss, neuroinflammation, and neurodegeneration in different kinds of dementia have been clarified by research into the neurobiology and pathophysiology of dementia. illness-modifying medicines that target pathological markers of dementia, like tau tangles, alpha-synuclein aggregates, amyloid-beta plaques, and TDP-43 inclusions, are being researched as possible targets to delay or stop the progression of the illness.

- Risk Factor Modification: A number of modifiable risk factors for dementia have been found by epidemiological studies. These include environmental factors (such as air pollution, traumatic brain injury), lifestyle factors (such as physical inactivity, smoking, unhealthy diet, and social isolation), and cardiovascular risk factors (such as hypertension, diabetes, obesity, and hypercholesterolemia). Reducing cardiovascular risk, changing one's lifestyle, and implementing environmental treatments are some of the risk factor-targeting strategies that show promise in preventing or postponing dementia and lowering the disease's worldwide impact.

- Interventional Trials: A number of pathological processes linked to the genesis of the disease, such as the synthesis and aggregation of amyloid-beta, the phosphorylation and aggregation of tau, neuroinflammation, synaptic dysfunction, and neuronal loss, are being targeted in clinical trials investigating disease-modifying therapies for dementia. The following therapeutic modalities are being researched: monoclonal antibodies that target tau and amyloid-beta; small molecule inhibitors that block the synthesis or aggregation of amyloid-beta; anti-inflammatory therapies; neuroprotective substances; and repurposed medications that may have the ability to change illness.

Optimistic Therapeutic Objectives

Preclinical and clinical research on dementia has identified a number of intriguing treatment targets that may be used to modify the disease, control symptoms, and maintain functional ability. The following are a few of the most promising treatment targets:

- Amyloid-beta and Tau: Since these proteins are essential to the etiology of tauopathies, including Alzheimer's disease, they are desirable targets for treatments that alter the course of the disease. The objective of clinical trials is to delay or stop the progression of the illness by pursuing strategies that target tau pathology, clear existing amyloid-beta plaques, reduce the synthesis of amyloid-beta, and prevent its aggregation.

- Neuroinflammation: Contributing to neurodegeneration, synaptic dysfunction, and neuronal injury, neuroinflammation is a major factor in the pathophysiology of dementia. It may be possible to reduce neuroinflammation and maintain neuronal function in dementia patients by using therapeutic strategies that target neuroinflammatory pathways, including as immune cell infiltration, cytokine signaling, and microglial activation.

- Synaptic Dysfunction: Impaired neural communication, synaptic plasticity, and cognitive function are the results of synaptic dysfunction, an early and noticeable hallmark of dementia. Potential methods for maintaining cognitive function and delaying the course of disease include therapeutic interventions targeted at improving synaptic function, encouraging synaptogenesis, and shielding synapses from degeneration.

- Neuroprotection and Neuroregeneration: In patients suffering from dementia, neuroprotective and neuroregenerative treatments seek to maintain preexisting neurons, encourage neuronal survival, and stimulate neurogenesis and synaptogenesis. The potential of neurotrophic factors, growth factors, stem cell-based medicines, and gene therapy approaches to safeguard neurons from harm, encourage neuronal repair, and reestablish cognitive function in dementia patients is being studied.

- Precision Medicine: This field of study aims to customize treatment plans based on patient variables such as disease stage, comorbidities, genetic profile, and biomarker profile. Personalized therapies aimed at certain pathogenic causes, molecular pathways, or dementia phenotypic traits show potential to maximize therapy responsiveness, reduce side effects, and enhance outcomes for dementia patients.

New Innovations and Technologies

New techniques for early dementia detection, diagnosis, monitoring, and treatment are being made possible by emerging technology and breakthroughs, which are revolutionizing dementia research and clinical care. The following are a few of the most exciting new developments and technology in dementia research:

- Artificial Intelligence and Machine Learning: Algorithms utilizing AI and machine learning have the capacity to evaluate extensive information, spot trends, forecast the course of disease, and create dementia diagnostic and prognostic models. AI-based tools are being created to improve dementia diagnosis precision, customize treatment regimens, and speed up dementia drug development. These technologies include neuroimaging analysis, biomarker discovery, cognitive evaluation, and drug discovery.

- Digital Health Technologies: By enabling real-time data collection, individualized interventions for dementia patients and their caregivers, and remote monitoring, digital health technologies—such as wearables, mobile apps, remote monitoring systems, and telehealth platforms—are revolutionizing the treatment of dementia. Care coordination, access to care, and the ability of individuals with dementia to control their condition are all being improved by the integration of digital health tools for cognitive testing, pharmaceutical management, behavioral monitoring, and caregiver support into clinical practice.

- Virtual and Augmented Reality: Technologies such as virtual reality (VR) and augmented reality (AR) provide people with dementia with immersive and interactive settings for cognitive training, rehabilitation, and sensory stimulation. The use of virtual reality (VR) in recollection therapy, exposure therapy, and spatial navigation training is being investigated as a non-pharmacological means of boosting social engagement, enhancing well-being, and improving cognitive performance in dementia patients.

- Neuroimaging Techniques: New developments in neuroimaging methods, including diffusion tensor imaging (DTI), functional magnetic resonance imaging (fMRI), positron emission tomography (PET), and magnetic resonance imaging (MRI), are shedding light on the anatomical, functional, and connectivity alterations in the brain linked to dementia. In order to visualize amyloid-beta, tau, neuroinflammation, and synaptic dysfunction in vivo and aid in early detection, differential diagnosis, and treatment monitoring in dementia patients, new imaging tracers, multimodal imaging approaches, and high-resolution imaging techniques are being developed.

- Biomarker Discovery Platforms: New biomarkers for dementia diagnosis, prognosis, and treatment response are being found thanks to biomarker discovery platforms that include mass spectrometry, proteomics, metabolomics, and genomes technologies. Personalized medicine approaches in dementia care are being made possible by the development of multiplex biomarker assays, liquid biopsy techniques, and point-of-care testing devices for the rapid, sensitive, and economical detection of dementia biomarkers in blood, saliva, urine, and cerebrospinal fluid.

In conclusion, a multidisciplinary strategy incorporating genetics, neurobiology, biomarkers, treatments, and technology characterizes research advances and future goals in dementia. Innovative interventions, cutting-edge technologies, and promising therapeutic targets have the potential to improve dementia patients' early diagnosis, care, and treatment, which will eventually improve the prognosis and quality of life for afflicted individuals and their families. To advance dementia research, translate scientific findings into clinical practice, and address the growing global challenge of dementia in the twenty-first century, collaboration among researchers, healthcare professionals, industry partners, policymakers, and patient advocates is imperative.

RESOURCES AND SUPPORT

For both the dementia patient and their caregiver, navigating the difficulties of dementia care can be daunting. Thankfully, there are plenty of tools and services available to offer guidance, help, and emotional support all throughout the dementia path. This section will look at local resources, dementia care resources, instructional materials, advocacy groups, and support groups.

Community Resources

By giving access to vital services, activities, and support networks, community resources play a critical role in supporting people with dementia and their carers. Typical community resources for dementia care include the following:

- Memory Clinics and Diagnostic Centers: These facilities provide thorough assessments, individualized treatment programs, and diagnostic tests to those with dementia and cognitive impairment. They also specialize in the examination, diagnosis, and management of memory disorders. Multidisciplinary teams of neurologists, geriatricians, neuropsychologists, social workers, and other medical experts with dementia care training are frequently seen at memory clinics.

- Aging and Disability Resource Centers (ADRCs): ADRCs help people with impairments, including those suffering from dementia, by offering information, support, and referrals. Care coordination, case management, long-term care planning, caregiver support, and access to community-based resources and activities are just a few of the many services provided by ADRCs.

- Adult Day Programs: During the day, adults with dementia can participate in structured activities, socializing, and supervision provided by adult day programs. This allows caregivers to take breaks, respond to their own needs, and continue working. Recreational activities, cognitive stimulation exercises, therapeutic interventions, and health monitoring services customized to the needs of dementia participants are all possible inclusions in adult day programs.

- Home Care Services: For people with dementia who want to continue living at home, home care services include assistance with both instrumental and daily living activities (ADLs and IADLs). Personal care support, medication administration, meal preparation, companionship, transportation, and caregiver respite care are a few examples of home care services.

- Caregiver Support Programs: These programs provide family caregivers of dementia patients with information, instruction, counseling, and respite care. These initiatives could consist of caregiver workshops, support groups, internet tools, and hotlines manned by qualified experts who give caregivers advice, information, and emotional support.

- Senior Centers and Community Centers: These establishments provide an array of activities and programs for senior citizens, especially those suffering from dementia. Exercise courses, music therapy, art therapy, memory groups, educational workshops, and social activities are a few examples of these programs. They are all intended to support socializing, cognitive stimulation, and overall wellbeing.

Educational Resources

When it comes to providing knowledge and information on dementia, its symptoms, diagnosis, treatment, and care, educational materials are essential in empowering people living with dementia, their carers, medical professionals, and the general public. Typical dementia education resources include the following:

- Brochures and Pamphlets: These materials offer succinct explanations of dementia, covering its causes, risk factors, symptoms, diagnosis, available treatments, and methods for providing care. To increase public awareness and educate the public on dementia, these materials are frequently disseminated in hospital settings, community centers, senior centers, and public libraries.

- Books and Manuals: Developed by professionals in the field of dementia care, these resources offer comprehensive knowledge and helpful guidance to those coping with dementia as well as their carers. End-of-life care, legal and financial planning, behavior control measures, communication skills, and coping mechanisms are a few possible topics. Books and manuals can be purchased online or borrowed from libraries. They are available in print and digital versions.

- Online Resources: People with dementia and their carers can find a plethora of information, resources, and support on websites, blogs, and online forums devoted to dementia care. Articles, videos, webinars, interactive tools, caregiver forums, and social media groups are a few examples of online resources that people can use to connect with others, exchange experiences, and get peer support.

- Caregiver Training Programs: These initiatives allow family caregivers of dementia patients access to formal instruction and skill development. These programs could consist of webinars, online classes, in-person seminars, and self-paced modules on subjects like legal and financial planning, behavioral management, communication skills, dementia awareness, and self-care practices.

- Public Awareness Campaigns: These initiatives increase knowledge about dementia and foster compassion, acceptance, and support for those who are impacted by the illness. Public service announcements, social media campaigns, neighborhood gatherings, and instructional materials given out in public areas, businesses, schools, and healthcare institutions are a few examples of these initiatives.

Advocacy Groups and Support Units

Advocacy organizations and support groups are essential in promoting awareness of the difficulties associated with dementia, fighting for the rights and needs of people living with the disease as well as their carers, and offering both practical and emotional support to those impacted by it. Several well-known dementia advocacy organizations and support groups include:

- Alzheimer's Association: The main voluntary health group for Alzheimer's research, care, and support is the Alzheimer's Association. For those who have Alzheimer's disease, their carers, and medical professionals, the association provides a wealth of information and support. These include advocacy campaigns, care consultations, support groups, helplines, and instructional materials.

- Alzheimer's Foundation of America: This national nonprofit organization is committed to giving people with Alzheimer's disease and their families the best possible care and support. The organization works to improve dementia care and increase public understanding of the illness by providing educational programs, caregiver support services, community outreach initiatives, and advocacy campaigns.

- Lewy Body Dementia Association: This nonprofit organization aims to assist those who have Lewy body dementia, as well as their family and caregivers. The organization provides Lewy body dementia research projects, caregiver assistance, support groups, online forums, and instructional materials.

The Frontotemporal Degeneration Association is a nonprofit organization whose mission is to enhance the quality of life for those who suffer from frontotemporal degeneration (FTD) and associated illnesses. In an effort to raise public knowledge and comprehension of FTD, the group provides caregiver support services, educational materials, financing for research, and lobbying opportunities.

- Online Support Groups: These online forums allow dementia patients and their carers a way to communicate, exchange stories, and get peer support from people who are aware of their struggles. Online support groups can be led by peer volunteers or qualified moderators and might concentrate on certain dementia kinds, caregiver responsibilities, or shared experiences.

To sum up, community-based initiatives, educational materials, advocacy groups, and support groups are just a few examples of the resources and support services available for dementia care. These organizations and groups are committed to assisting those impacted by dementia and their carers with information, support, and emotional support. Through the use of these tools and services, people who are caring for someone with dementia and their carers can connect with others going through similar experiences, get emotional support, and discover useful assistance, all of which can improve their quality of life and overall wellbeing as the dementia process progresses.

PERSONAL STORIES AND REFLECTIONS

A unique view into the life experiences of people impacted by dementia, including those who have been diagnosed with the illness and their carers, is provided via personal narratives and reflections. Readers can develop a deeper knowledge of the difficulties, victories, and feelings related to dementia by reading these narratives, which offer compassion, inspiration, and empathy. This area will cover the viewpoints of those who have dementia, the experiences and observations of caregivers, and motivational tales of resiliency and optimism.

Views from Persons Affected by Dementia

Personal accounts from people who are dealing with dementia provide priceless insights into their feelings, ideas, and experiences as they deal with the difficulties posed by the illness. Even while dementia can cause cognitive decline and functional restrictions, people who have the disease frequently nevertheless have a vibrant inner life that is full of memories, feelings, and wants. Their experiences demonstrate how crucial person-centered care, respect, and autonomy are in helping people with dementia lead purposeful lives.

Being diagnosed with dementia may be a frightening and transformative experience for many people. Shock, denial, anxiety, and future uncertainty are possible initial reactions. But as time goes on, a lot of people with dementia learn to accept their diagnosis, reinterpret who they are, and concentrate on the things they can still achieve and enjoy right now.

Some dementia sufferers decide to openly discuss their experiences in order to raise awareness and promote acceptance as well as assistance for those who are coping with the illness. Through their writing, art, advocacy work, and speaking engagements, they fight stigma, dispel myths, and advance knowledge of dementia as a medical diagnosis as opposed to a human failing.

Experiences and Perspectives of Caregivers

Caregivers are essential to the lives of people with dementia because they offer them practical, emotional, and physical support at every stage of the illness. Their perspectives and experiences provide insightful lessons on the challenges, joys, and complexities of providing dementia care for a loved one. Caregiver testimonies emphasize the value of empathy, forbearance, and fortitude in overcoming the day-to-day difficulties associated with providing dementia care.

An array of feelings, such as grief, guilt, frustration, and tiredness, are frequently experienced by caregivers as they see a loved one's condition worsen and take on more and more caregiving duties. Many caregivers suffer from burnout, depression, and social isolation as a result of their constant battle to strike a balance between their personal needs and well-being and the obligations of providing care.

Despite the difficulties, a lot of caregivers find purpose and happiness in their work, treasured times of closeness, love, and connection with their loved ones suffering from dementia. Utilizing their resourcefulness and tenacity, they devise innovative approaches to problem-solving, communication, and involvement as they negotiate the intricacies of dementia care.

Support networks—which include friends, family, support groups, and expert services—are essential to maintaining the resilience and general well-being of caregivers. Fostering relationships with like-minded individuals, exchanging narratives, and requesting assistance when required can furnish caregivers with the resilience and backing they require to persist in their caregiving expedition.

Inspirational Narratives of Fortitude and Hope

Stories of fortitude, bravery, and optimism among the difficulties of dementia encourage us to realize the possibility of development, transformation, and connection even in the face of hardship. Inspirational tales of people with dementia and the people who care for them serve as a reminder of the human spirit's resiliency, flexibility, and capacity for love.

Despite their cognitive limitations, some people with dementia show incredible creativity, insight, and wisdom, defying assumptions and preconceptions. They continue to challenge stereotypes about what it means to live with dementia by sharing their distinct perspectives, talents, and contributions with the world through writing, music, art, and other forms of expression.

As they traverse the highs and lows of the dementia journey and find moments of happiness, laughter, and connection despite the difficulties, caregivers also exhibit resilience and fortitude. Their tales of love, commitment, and sacrifice encourage us to value the strong ties of friendship, family, and community that help us get through the difficult times in life.

Remarkable tales of tenacity and optimism serve as a reminder that dementia is merely a new chapter in life's journey rather than its conclusion. We can help people with dementia and those who care for them live with dignity, meaning, and purpose by embracing compassion, empathy, and understanding. We can also celebrate the resiliency of the human spirit and help them to treasure each moment of life.

Ultimately, anecdotes and introspective pieces about dementia provide significant understanding of the range of feelings, experiences, and viewpoints held by those who have the illness as well as those who care for them. People with dementia and those who care for them dispel misconceptions, shed light on the intricacies of the dementia journey, and encourage compassion, optimism, and resilience in others via their personal stories. We can improve our knowledge about dementia, encourage empathy and compassion, and create a more accepting and encouraging community for everyone impacted by the illness by paying attention to and respecting these individual stories.

CONCLUSION

While having dementia comes with its own set of difficulties, it also gives chances for development, resilience, and connection. As we come to the end of our investigation into dementia care, it's critical to emphasize that people with dementia may lead meaningful lives if they are given the support, understanding, and empowerment they need.

People suffering from dementia should first and foremost acknowledge their intrinsic value, humanity, and dignity. Dementia is only one part of your path; it does not define who you are. Regardless of any cognitive changes you may be going through, you still have a lifetime's worth of experiences, wisdom, and talents that should be acknowledged.

It's critical to keep your attention on your abilities rather than wallowing in your shortcomings or losses. Even though dementia may cause cognitive difficulties, there are still a lot of areas in life where you can succeed and feel satisfied. There are so many things you can do to bring joy and connection into your life, like being creative, taking in the beauty of nature, spending time with loved ones, or just taking it moment by moment.

Look for resources and assistance to help you deal with the difficulties caused by dementia. On your trip, you are not alone; a multitude of individuals and groups are prepared to provide support, direction, and camaraderie. Reaching out for assistance can have a big impact on your quality of life, whether it's through connection with healthcare professionals that specialize in dementia care, joining a support group, or using dementia-friendly services.

Speak up for both yourself and other dementia sufferers. Your opinion counts, and you can influence laws, plans of action, and other initiatives that will better serve the needs of those who are caring for loved ones who have dementia. Sharing your experience, bringing attention to the issue, and vocalizing opposition to prejudice and stigma will help create a society that is more accepting and encouraging to all.

Above all, keep in mind that, despite any cognitive changes you may be going through, you are deserving of love, respect, and dignity. You have the right to live your life to the fullest, supported by people who care about you and who think highly of you.

My dear friends, having dementia may come with difficulties, but it does not lessen your value or the quality of your life. Every single one of you has a distinct tale to tell, full with moments, encounters, and successes deserving of recognition and celebration.

Your diagnosis does not define you. Beyond that, you are so much more. You possess bravery, resiliency, and the ability to overcome any obstacles that may arise. You are capable of handling this path with dignity and grace because you are strong and powerful enough.

Yes, there are definitely going to be happy, loving, and connected moments mixed in with times of irritation, uncertainty, and confusion. Treasure those times. Treasure them. Allow them to lead the way when things get tough.

Be in the company of loving and supportive people. Rely on them as required. They are prepared to lend you a shoulder to cry on, a listening ear, or a helpful hand.

Recall that you are not traveling alone. Beside you, prepared to walk this route together, is a large community of people with dementia, caregivers, medical experts, and advocates.

So, my darling friends, greet every day with bravery and hope. Embrace happiness in the little things. Tell us about your experiences. Tell the truth what you know. And understand that exactly as you are, you are loved, treasured, and respected.

By working together, we can make a world in which people who have dementia are accepted for who they are and are seen, heard, and valued. Let's unify in our commitment to promoting empowerment, dignity, and compassion for all.

You're not by yourself. You deserve it. You are cherished. You are also capable of leading a happy, meaningful, and purposeful life.

Have confidence in yourself. Have faith in your abilities. And never lose sight of the amazing influence you have on the world.